# BEYOND THE DIAGNOSIS

## THRIVING WITH ADDISON'S DISEASE

## DR. EMMANUEL DEAN

# Copyright

**No part of this book should be copied, reproduced without the author's permission © 2024**

# Table of content


BEYOND THE DIAGNOSIS ..................................1

THRIVING WITH ADDISON'S DISEASE ..................1

DR. EMMANUEL DEAN ..................................1

Copyright ..................................................2

INTRODUCTION..........................................5

CHAPTER 1 ................................................9

UNDERSTANDING ADDISON DISEASE ..................9

Causes and Risk Factors of Addison's Disease:10

Risk Factors..............................................15

Anatomy of the Adrenal Glands ..................18

Chapter Two ............................................26

Symptoms and Diagnosis of Addison's Disease ...26

Early Signs and Symptoms of Addison's
Disease ..................................................27

Diagnosing Addison's Disease ..................31

Differential Diagnosis of Addison's Disease...33

Chapter three ..........................................38

Types of Addison's Disease..........................38

Primary vs. Secondary Addison's Disease......38

Atypical Forms of Addison's Disease ............42

Chapter four ............................................45

Treatment Options for Addison's Disease ...........45

Hormone Replacement Therapy in Addison's
Disease ......................................................46

Medications in Addison's Disease .................48

Individualized Treatment Plans in Addison's
Disease ......................................................50

Chapter five ....................................................53

Managing Daily Life with Addison's Disease ........53

Lifestyle Adjustments for Well-being in
Addison's Disease .......................................54

Exercise and Physical Activity in Addison's
Disease: ....................................................57

Other important lifestyle adjustments ..........59

Chapter six ....................................................62

Complications and Associated Conditions in
Addison's Disease ............................................62

Adrenal Crisis in Addison's Disease ..............63

Autoimmune Disorders in the Context of
Addison's Disease .......................................65

Mental Health Considerations in Addison's
Disease ......................................................67

Chapter seven .................................................70

Medical Monitoring in Addison's Disease...........70

Blood Tests and Monitoring Parameters in
Addison's Disease ......................................73

Emergency Preparedness in Addison's Disease76

Chapter eight ..................................................79

Support Systems in Addison's Disease................79

Support Groups and Communities in Addison's Disease ..................................80
Psychological Support in Addison's Disease ..83
Educating Family and Friends about Addison's Disease ..................................85
Chapter nine ..................................87
Research and Future Developments in Addison's Disease..................................87
Current Research in Addison's Disease .........88
Potential Breakthroughs in Addison's Disease90
Chapter 10 ..................................94
Personal Stories and Perspectives .....................94
True life story from a patient .................96
Caregiver Perspectives in Addison's Disease .98
Chapter eleven..................................102
Appendix..................................102
Glossary of Terms in Addison's Disease and Endocrinology..................................102
Additional Resources for Addison's Disease Support and Information..................................106
Pharmacy Support Programs..................................108
Conclusion ..................................110

# INTRODUCTION

Addison's Disease is a rare but significant medical condition characterized by the insufficient production of hormones by the adrenal glands, leading to a range of symptoms affecting various systems in the body. This introduction will provide an in-depth exploration of the definition of Addison's Disease, offering clarity on the condition's nature and impact. Additionally, we'll delve into a historical overview to understand how our understanding and management of this disorder have evolved over time.

**Definition of Addison's Disease:**
Addison's Disease, also known as primary adrenal insufficiency or hypoadrenalism, is a disorder that results from the adrenal glands' inability to produce an adequate amount of cortisol and, in some cases, aldosterone. These hormones play pivotal roles in regulating metabolism, blood pressure, and the body's response to stress. When the adrenal glands fail to produce sufficient amounts of these hormones, it can lead to a myriad of symptoms and complications.

The condition is typically caused by an autoimmune response, where the body's immune system mistakenly attacks and damages the adrenal glands. Other causes may include infections, cancer, or genetic factors. Addison's Disease can occur at any age and affects both genders equally. It often progresses slowly, and symptoms may not manifest until a significant percentage of adrenal function is lost.

**Historical Overview:**
The history of Addison's Disease is intertwined with the discovery and understanding of the adrenal glands and their functions. Named after the renowned British physician Thomas Addison, who first described the condition in 1855, Addison's Disease gained recognition as a distinct medical entity.

Thomas Addison's meticulous observations of patients with a specific set of symptoms, including fatigue, weight loss, and skin hyperpigmentation, led to the identification of adrenal insufficiency. He associated these symptoms with structural changes in the adrenal glands, marking a crucial milestone in the history of endocrinology.

Throughout the late 19th and early 20th centuries, medical pioneers expanded on Addison's initial observations. Researchers like William Osler and C. E. Brown-Séquard furthered our understanding of adrenal function and the significance of adrenal hormones.

Advancements in medical technology and research methodologies in the latter half of the 20th century contributed to a more nuanced comprehension of Addison's Disease. The identification of the autoimmune nature of the condition and the development of diagnostic tools, such as the adrenocorticotropic hormone (ACTH) stimulation test, enhanced our ability to diagnose and manage the disorder.

In recent decades, genetic studies have provided valuable insights into the hereditary aspects of Addison's Disease, offering potential avenues for early detection and personalized treatment strategies. The integration of molecular biology and advanced imaging techniques continues to refine our understanding of adrenal function and dysfunction.

The historical evolution of Addison's Disease reflects the collaborative efforts of physicians, researchers, and scientists across different eras. From its initial recognition by Thomas Addison to contemporary genetic investigations, the journey has been marked by a commitment to unraveling the complexities of adrenal insufficiency and improving the lives of those affected.

In summary, Addison's Disease is a complex endocrine disorder with a rich historical background. Understanding its definition and historical context lays the foundation for a comprehensive exploration of this condition, encompassing its clinical manifestations, diagnosis, and contemporary management approaches.

# CHAPTER 1

# UNDERSTANDING ADDISON

# DISEASE

Understanding Addison's Disease requires a comprehensive grasp of its multifaceted nature. This rare condition arises from the malfunction of the adrenal glands, which sit atop the kidneys and produce vital hormones like cortisol and aldosterone. The primary cause often involves autoimmune responses, where the body mistakenly attacks and damages these crucial glands.

To delve deeper, one must explore the intricate anatomy of the adrenal glands and the intricate web of hormonal regulation they orchestrate. Cortisol, often termed the "stress hormone," influences metabolism, immune response, and the body's reaction to stressors. Aldosterone regulates electrolyte balance and plays a pivotal role in maintaining blood pressure. Furthermore, comprehending the pathophysiology of Addison's Disease unveils the gradual deterioration of adrenal function. This breakdown, whether due to autoimmune processes, infections, or genetic factors, leads to a cascade of symptoms. Early signs may include fatigue, weight loss, and skin hyperpigmentation, reflecting the disruption in hormonal equilibrium. In essence, understanding Addison's Disease involves navigating the intricacies of adrenal gland function, recognizing the diverse factors triggering its onset, and appreciating the far-reaching consequences of hormonal imbalance on various physiological processes. This foundational knowledge lays the groundwork for a more profound exploration of diagnosis, treatment, and holistic management strategies.

## Causes and Risk Factors of Addison's Disease:

Addison's Disease, a rare but significant disorder, stems from a delicate interplay of genetic, autoimmune, and environmental factors that converge to disrupt the normal functioning of the adrenal glands. As we embark on an exploration of its causes and risk factors, we delve into the intricate mechanisms triggering this condition and the diverse array of elements that may contribute to its onset.

- ❖ **Autoimmune Processes:** At the forefront of Addison's Disease causation lies autoimmune dysfunction. In approximately 70-90% of cases, the body's immune system mistakenly perceives the adrenal glands as foreign entities and launches an attack. This autoimmune assault leads to inflammation and damage to the adrenal cortex, the outer layer responsible for producing cortisol and aldosterone. The specific triggers initiating this autoimmune response remain elusive, although genetic predispositions likely play a crucial role. Autoimmune adrenalitis, the term used to describe this immune-mediated damage, gradually impairs adrenal function, setting the stage for the characteristic insufficiency observed in Addison's Disease.

- ❖ **Infections and Tuberculosis:** Infections, particularly those affecting the adrenal glands directly, can contribute to the development of Addison's Disease. Tuberculosis, historically a prominent cause, can infiltrate the adrenal glands, leading to inflammation and scarring. The resulting damage impedes the glands' ability to produce hormones adequately. While tuberculosis-related Addison's Disease has become less prevalent in regions with improved tuberculosis control, infectious agents can still trigger adrenal insufficiency. Fungal infections, such as histoplasmosis and coccidioidomycosis, also pose a risk, emphasizing the diverse infectious etiologies associated with this condition.

❖ **Genetic Factors:** Genetic predisposition plays a pivotal role in Addison's Disease, although the precise genetic mechanisms remain complex. Studies suggest a familial clustering of autoimmune diseases, indicating a hereditary component. Specific genetic markers associated with increased susceptibility to autoimmune adrenalitis have been identified, shedding light on the hereditary aspects of this disorder. The Human Leukocyte Antigen (HLA) system, a group of genes involved in immune system regulation, is implicated in the genetic susceptibility to autoimmune disorders, including Addison's Disease. Familial forms of Addison's Disease have been documented, emphasizing the importance of genetic factors in shaping an individual's vulnerability to adrenal insufficiency.

❖ **Adrenal Hemorrhage:** Adrenal hemorrhage, a rare but noteworthy cause, can precipitate Addison's Disease. This often occurs in the context of severe infections, trauma, or complications during childbirth. The sudden bleeding into the adrenal glands compromises their structural integrity, impairing hormone production. Neonatal adrenal hemorrhage, occurring in newborns, is a distinct entity associated with perinatal stress and is a recognized cause of adrenal insufficiency in this population.

❖ **Medications and Surgical Removal:** Certain medications, especially those used in the treatment of autoimmune disorders, may inadvertently trigger adrenal insufficiency. Long-term use of glucocorticoids, such as prednisone, can suppress the adrenal glands' natural hormone production. Abrupt cessation of these medications can lead to adrenal crisis, emphasizing the delicate balance required in managing autoimmune conditions without compromising adrenal function. Additionally, surgical removal of adrenal glands for conditions like tumors or cancer can result in Addison's Disease. This scenario necessitates careful consideration of hormonal replacement therapy to mitigate the impact of adrenal gland removal.

- ❖ **Amyloidosis:** Amyloidosis, a rare condition characterized by the abnormal deposition of protein aggregates (amyloids) in various tissues, can affect the adrenal glands. When amyloids accumulate in the adrenal cortex, they disrupt normal glandular function, contributing to adrenal insufficiency. While amyloidosis is an uncommon cause of Addison's Disease, its inclusion underscores the diverse pathogenic pathways leading to adrenal dysfunction.

- ❖ **Idiopathic Addison's Disease:** In a subset of cases, Addison's Disease may occur without a clear identifiable cause, termed idiopathic adrenal insufficiency. This designation is often assigned when the etiology remains elusive despite thorough investigation. The idiopathic variant highlights the gaps in our current understanding of all potential triggers and emphasizes the need for ongoing research to unravel the complexities of adrenal dysfunction.

## Risk Factors

Beyond the specific causes, certain risk factors increase the likelihood of developing Addison's Disease or experiencing adrenal insufficiency. These risk factors provide valuable insights for clinicians in identifying individuals who may benefit from closer monitoring or proactive measures.

- **Age and Gender:** Addison's Disease can manifest at any age, but it often becomes clinically apparent in individuals between the ages of 30 and 50. While gender distribution is generally equal, some studies suggest a slight predilection for females. The reasons behind age and gender associations remain topics of ongoing research, with hormonal and immunological factors being explored.

- **Family History:** A family history of autoimmune disorders, particularly those involving the endocrine system, increases the risk of developing Addison's Disease. The shared genetic susceptibility within families underscores the importance of considering familial medical histories in assessing an individual's predisposition to adrenal insufficiency.

- **Autoimmune Disorders:** Individuals with pre-existing autoimmune conditions, such as type 1 diabetes, autoimmune thyroid diseases (like Hashimoto's thyroiditis), or vitiligo, have an elevated risk of developing Addison's Disease. The co-occurrence of multiple autoimmune disorders highlights shared underlying immunological mechanisms contributing to various endocrine dysfunctions.

- **Infections and Trauma:** Previous infections, especially those involving the adrenal glands, may increase the likelihood of subsequent adrenal insufficiency. Similarly, trauma or injury to the adrenal glands, whether through accidents or surgical procedures, poses a potential risk factor. Recognizing these historical factors can aid in the clinical assessment of individuals with suspected adrenal dysfunction.

- **Medication Use:** The prolonged and high-dose use of glucocorticoid medications, whether for autoimmune diseases or other inflammatory conditions, heightens the risk of adrenal suppression. Clinicians must carefully manage these medications to balance therapeutic benefits with the potential risk of inducing adrenal insufficiency.

- **Pregnancy**: Pregnancy places additional stress on the endocrine system, and women with Addison's Disease may need adjustments in their hormonal replacement therapy during pregnancy. Adequate monitoring and collaboration between obstetricians and endocrinologists are crucial to ensuring optimal outcomes for both the mother and the developing fetus.

Understanding the causes and risk factors illuminates the diverse pathways leading to adrenal insufficiency, guiding clinicians in diagnosis, treatment, and preventive strategies.

# Anatomy of the Adrenal Glands

The adrenal glands, two small glands nestled atop the kidneys, play a pivotal role in maintaining homeostasis within the human body. To comprehend the intricacies of adrenal function and the significance of these walnut-sized glands, a closer look at their anatomy is essential.

## Adrenal Cortex

**Layers of Hormonal Synthesis:** The adrenal glands consist of two distinct regions: the outer adrenal cortex and the inner adrenal medulla. The adrenal cortex, responsible for the synthesis of vital hormones, is further divided into three layers: the zona glomerulosa, zona fasciculata, and zona reticularis.

**Zona Glomerulosa:** Located on the outermost layer, this region primarily produces mineralocorticoids, with aldosterone being the key hormone. Aldosterone regulates electrolyte balance, particularly the levels of sodium and potassium, contributing to blood pressure regulation.

**Zona Fasciculata:** Situated beneath the zona glomerulosa, the zona fasciculata synthesizes glucocorticoids, predominantly cortisol. Cortisol influences metabolism, immune response, and the body's ability to cope with stress. Its intricate regulatory role extends to glucose metabolism and anti-inflammatory processes.

**Zona Reticularis:** Positioned adjacent to the medulla, the zona reticularis synthesizes androgens, including dehydroepiandrosterone (DHEA) and androstenedione. While these androgens are present in both males and females, their role in adrenal function is more pronounced in females, contributing to the overall endocrine balance.

**Adrenal Medulla**

The Epicenter of Catecholamines: Deeper within the adrenal glands lies the adrenal medulla, an integral part of the sympathetic nervous system. Specialized cells called chromaffin cells in the medulla synthesize and release catecholamines, including adrenaline (epinephrine) and noradrenaline (norepinephrine). These hormones rapidly respond to stressors, initiating the "fight or flight" response. They elevate heart rate, increase blood flow to muscles, and prepare the body for immediate action.

## Blood Supply and Structural Considerations

The adrenal glands boast a rich blood supply, receiving blood from multiple arteries, including the superior, middle, and inferior adrenal arteries. This profuse vascularization underscores the glands' importance in systemic regulation. Structurally, each adrenal gland is composed of an outer capsule, surrounding the cortex and medulla, and an inner adrenal medulla. The glands' position atop the kidneys ensures close proximity to vital blood vessels and facilitates efficient hormonal secretion directly into the bloodstream.

## Regulation of Adrenal Function

The synthesis and release of hormones from the adrenal glands are tightly regulated by complex feedback mechanisms. The hypothalamus, a region in the brain, releases corticotropin-releasing hormone (CRH), which signals the pituitary gland to produce adrenocorticotropic hormone (ACTH). ACTH, in turn, stimulates the adrenal cortex to secrete cortisol and other corticosteroids. This intricate regulatory loop, known as the hypothalamic-pituitary-adrenal

(HPA) axis, ensures a finely tuned hormonal balance within the body.

**Adrenal Glands in Stress Response**
The adrenal glands' crucial role in the stress response is particularly evident during acute and chronic stress. In challenging situations, the sympathetic nervous system prompts the release of catecholamines from the adrenal medulla, initiating rapid physiological changes. Simultaneously, the adrenal cortex releases cortisol to sustain the body's response to prolonged stressors, modulating metabolism and immune function.

The anatomy of the adrenal glands unveils a remarkable orchestration of hormonal synthesis and regulation that influences nearly every aspect of the body's functioning. From the mineralocorticoids of the zona glomerulosa to the androgens of the zona reticularis and the catecholamines of the adrenal medulla, these glands are integral to maintaining homeostasis. The interconnected layers of the adrenal cortex and the dynamic responses orchestrated by the adrenal medulla illustrate the elegance of this endocrine powerhouse. A deeper understanding of adrenal anatomy lays the foundation for unraveling the complexities of adrenal disorders, such as Addison's Disease, and underscores the vital role these glands play in our overall health.

**Pathophysiology of Addison's Disease**
Addison's Disease, characterized by adrenal insufficiency, has a pathophysiology intricately linked to the malfunction of the adrenal glands. Understanding the underlying processes sheds light on how this disorder manifests and progresses.

- **Autoimmune Destruction of Adrenal Tissue:** In the majority of Addison's cases, autoimmune processes lie at the heart of the pathophysiology. The immune system, typically a defender against foreign invaders, turns hostile and erroneously targets the adrenal glands. Specifically, the outer layer of the adrenal glands, known as the adrenal cortex, becomes the battleground. This autoimmune assault leads to chronic inflammation and gradual destruction of adrenal tissue, particularly the cells responsible for producing cortisol and aldosterone.

- **Impact on Hormone Production:** The primary consequence of autoimmune destruction is the impaired synthesis and secretion of essential hormones. Cortisol, a glucocorticoid crucial for metabolic regulation and stress response, is significantly reduced. Aldosterone, a mineralocorticoid pivotal for maintaining electrolyte balance and blood pressure, also experiences a marked decline. This hormonal deficit results in a cascade of physiological disruptions, affecting various organs and systems throughout the body.

- **Progressive Nature of the Disease:** Addison's Disease often progresses slowly, and symptoms may not become apparent until a substantial percentage of adrenal function is compromised. As autoimmune processes persist, the adrenal glands' ability to produce hormones diminishes, leading to a state of chronic insufficiency. The gradual decline in hormone levels underscores the insidious nature of the disorder, making early detection and intervention challenging.

- **Adrenal Crisis:** In some cases, Addison's Disease may manifest acutely in the form of an adrenal crisis. This life-threatening situation occurs when stressors, such as infections, trauma, or surgery, overwhelm the compromised adrenal glands. The sudden demand for increased cortisol and aldosterone exceeds the glands' diminished capacity, resulting in a rapid deterioration of health. Adrenal crisis is a medical emergency, requiring prompt intervention with hormone replacement therapy and supportive measures to stabilize the individual.

- **Genetic and Non-Autoimmune Causes:** While autoimmune mechanisms dominate, there are instances where Addison's Disease arises from genetic factors or non-autoimmune causes. Genetic predisposition may contribute to an individual's susceptibility to autoimmune adrenalitis. Additionally, infections, tuberculosis historically being notable, and adrenal hemorrhage due to trauma or other underlying conditions can disrupt adrenal function and lead to adrenal insufficiency.

- **Diagnostic Challenges:** Diagnosing Addison's Disease can be challenging due to its gradual onset and nonspecific symptoms. The pathophysiological processes within the adrenal glands may be underway long before clinical manifestations become evident. The identification of specific autoantibodies associated with autoimmune adrenalitis, such as anti-21-hydroxylase antibodies, aids in confirming the autoimmune nature of the disorder and supporting the diagnosis. The pathophysiology of Addison's Disease is a dynamic interplay of autoimmune destruction, hormonal deficiencies, and the progressive deterioration of adrenal function. Understanding these processes is pivotal for timely diagnosis, initiation of hormone replacement therapy, and management of potential complications.

# Chapter Two

# Symptoms and Diagnosis of

# Addison's Disease

Addison's Disease manifests through a spectrum of symptoms, often nonspecific and insidious in onset. Early recognition of these signs is crucial for timely intervention. Common symptoms include fatigue, weight loss, and hyperpigmentation, particularly in sun-exposed areas. Muscle weakness, low blood pressure, and salt cravings may also arise due to aldosterone deficiency, impacting electrolyte balance.

Diagnosing Addison's Disease involves a comprehensive approach. Clinical suspicion arises when patients present with a constellation of symptoms and risk factors. Laboratory tests measuring cortisol and adrenocorticotropic hormone (ACTH) levels serve as initial indicators.

In Addison's, cortisol levels are typically low, while ACTH levels are elevated due to the lack of negative feedback on the pituitary gland. Further confirmation often involves the cosyntropin stimulation test, where synthetic ACTH is administered, and cortisol response is measured. Imaging studies, such as CT scans, may reveal atrophy or calcification of the adrenal glands, supporting the diagnosis. Recognition of specific autoantibodies associated with autoimmune adrenalitis aids in confirming the autoimmune nature of the disorder, providing valuable insights for tailored management strategies. The intricate interplay of clinical findings and diagnostic tests allows healthcare professionals to unravel the complex puzzle of Addison's Disease and initiate appropriate therapeutic interventions.

## Early Signs and Symptoms of Addison's Disease

Addison's Disease, often referred to as primary adrenal insufficiency, presents a myriad of early signs and symptoms that, in their subtlety, can pose diagnostic challenges. Recognizing these initial manifestations is crucial for timely intervention and the prevention of potential complications.

◆ **Fatigue and Weakness:** One of the hallmark early symptoms of Addison's Disease is persistent fatigue and generalized weakness. Individuals may find themselves chronically tired, even after adequate rest, and experience a noticeable decline in stamina. This fatigue results from the insufficient production of cortisol, a hormone crucial for maintaining energy levels and metabolic balance.

◆ **Weight Loss:** Unintentional weight loss is another common early sign. Adrenal insufficiency can lead to decreased appetite and alterations in metabolism, causing individuals to shed pounds without apparent cause. The weight loss is often gradual but can be significant over time.

◆ **Gastrointestinal Distress:** Early stages of Addison's Disease may manifest with gastrointestinal symptoms, including nausea, vomiting, and abdominal discomfort. These symptoms arise from the disruption of normal digestive processes due to hormonal imbalances, particularly the deficiency of cortisol.

◆ **Hyperpigmentation:** Hyperpigmentation, or darkening of the skin, is a distinctive feature of Addison's Disease. This occurs due to elevated levels of adrenocorticotropic hormone (ACTH), which stimulates melanin production. The hyperpigmentation is most prominent in sun-exposed areas, such as the face, neck, and hands. Individuals may develop a characteristic bronzed or tanned appearance.

◆ **Hypotension and Dizziness:** Adrenal insufficiency can lead to low blood pressure (hypotension), contributing to dizziness and lightheadedness. The lack of aldosterone, a hormone responsible for maintaining sodium and potassium balance, affects fluid regulation and blood pressure.

◆ **Salt Cravings and Dehydration:** Aldosterone deficiency can result in an imbalance of electrolytes, leading to salt cravings. Individuals may find themselves drawn to salty foods as the body attempts to compensate for the electrolyte imbalance. Additionally, impaired water and salt retention can contribute to dehydration, amplifying feelings of weakness and dizziness.

◆ **Muscle and Joint Pain:** Early stages of Addison's Disease may involve muscle and joint pain. This discomfort can be attributed to the impact of cortisol deficiency on inflammation and the body's ability to cope with physical stressors.

◆ **Hypoglycemia:** Cortisol plays a crucial role in regulating glucose metabolism. In Addison's Disease, decreased cortisol levels can lead to hypoglycemia (low blood sugar), resulting in symptoms such as shakiness, irritability, and confusion.

◆ **Mood Changes:** Hormonal imbalances in Addison's Disease can affect mood and mental well-being. Individuals may experience irritability, anxiety, or depression, reflecting the broader impact of adrenal dysfunction on the central nervous system.

Recognizing these early signs is challenging due to their nonspecific nature, often resembling symptoms of other medical conditions. A comprehensive clinical assessment, coupled with laboratory tests measuring cortisol and ACTH levels, aids in differentiating Addison's Disease from other disorders.

## Diagnosing Addison's Disease

Diagnosing Addison's Disease demands a systematic approach, considering its insidious onset and diverse, often nonspecific, symptoms. The process involves a combination of clinical evaluation, laboratory tests, and imaging studies to unravel the complex web of adrenal dysfunction.

⬥ **Clinical Assessment:** The diagnostic journey often begins with a thorough clinical assessment. Healthcare professionals explore the patient's medical history, paying close attention to symptoms such as fatigue, weight loss, gastrointestinal disturbances, hyperpigmentation, and episodes of hypotension or dehydration. A detailed family history is also crucial, as Addison's Disease may exhibit familial clustering, highlighting potential genetic predispositions.

✧ **Laboratory Tests:** Key laboratory tests serve as pivotal indicators in the diagnostic process. Initial assessments include measuring serum cortisol levels and adrenocorticotropic hormone (ACTH) levels. In Addison's Disease, cortisol levels are typically low, while ACTH levels are elevated due to the lack of negative feedback on the pituitary gland. To further confirm adrenal insufficiency, clinicians often perform the cosyntropin stimulation test. In this test, a synthetic form of ACTH (cosyntropin) is administered, and the patient's cortisol response is measured. In individuals with Addison's Disease, cortisol levels exhibit a muted or absent response, highlighting the compromised adrenal function.

✧ **Autoantibody Testing:** Given the autoimmune nature of most Addison's cases, specific autoantibody testing is valuable. The presence of autoantibodies, particularly anti-21-hydroxylase antibodies, supports the diagnosis of autoimmune adrenalitis. These antibodies target an enzyme involved in cortisol synthesis, providing a distinctive marker for autoimmune destruction of the adrenal glands.

✧ **Imaging Studies:** Imaging studies, such as computed tomography (CT) scans, can offer insights into the structural integrity of the adrenal glands. In Addison's Disease, atrophy or calcification of the adrenal glands may be visible. While imaging studies are not diagnostic on their own, they provide valuable information supporting the overall clinical picture.

✧ **Electrolyte and Metabolic Panel:** Addison's Disease often leads to electrolyte imbalances, particularly decreased levels of sodium and increased levels of potassium. Conducting a comprehensive electrolyte and metabolic panel aids in assessing these imbalances and their impact on overall health.

In conclusion, diagnosing Addison's Disease involves a meticulous blend of clinical acumen, laboratory assessments, and imaging studies.

## Differential Diagnosis of Addison's Disease

The symptoms of Addison's Disease, while distinctive, can overlap with those of various other medical conditions, necessitating a thorough differential diagnosis. Distinguishing Addison's from other disorders with similar presentations is crucial for accurate treatment and management.

- **Secondary Adrenal Insufficiency:** Secondary adrenal insufficiency, unlike primary adrenal insufficiency in Addison's Disease, results from dysfunction in the pituitary gland or hypothalamus. Tumors, infections, or other structural issues in these regions can compromise the production of adrenocorticotropic hormone (ACTH), leading to reduced cortisol synthesis. Differentiating between primary and secondary adrenal insufficiency is pivotal, as the management approaches differ.

- **Adrenal Tumors:** Tumors affecting the adrenal glands, such as adrenal adenomas or carcinomas, may present with symptoms similar to Addison's Disease. These tumors can disrupt normal adrenal function, causing hormonal imbalances. Imaging studies, including CT scans, help identify the presence and characteristics of adrenal tumors.

- **Pituitary Disorders:** Disorders affecting the pituitary gland, such as pituitary tumors or

Sheehan's syndrome, can impact ACTH production. Reduced ACTH levels subsequently lead to insufficient stimulation of cortisol production by the adrenal glands. Evaluating pituitary function and hormonal levels aids in distinguishing these disorders from Addison's Disease.

- **Hypothyroidism**: Hypothyroidism, characterized by an underactive thyroid, shares some symptoms with Addison's Disease, including fatigue, weight loss, and mood changes. A comprehensive thyroid function panel helps assess thyroid hormone levels, aiding in the differentiation of these endocrine disorders.

- **Diabetes Mellitus:** Both Addison's Disease and diabetes mellitus can manifest with weight loss, fatigue, and gastrointestinal disturbances. Differentiating between the two involves assessing blood glucose levels and evaluating the specific symptoms associated with each condition.

- **Gastrointestinal Disorders:** Disorders such as celiac disease, inflammatory bowel disease (IBD), or chronic infections can present with gastrointestinal symptoms akin to those observed in Addison's Disease. Clinical evaluation, along with specific tests for these gastrointestinal conditions, assists in the differential diagnosis.

- **Chronic Fatigue Syndrome:** Chronic fatigue syndrome shares the symptom of persistent fatigue with Addison's Disease. However, the absence of adrenal-specific hormonal imbalances in chronic fatigue syndrome helps distinguish between the two conditions.

- **Electrolyte Imbalance:** Conditions leading to electrolyte imbalances, such as renal disorders or certain medications, may cause symptoms resembling those seen in Addison's Disease. Comprehensive metabolic panels and detailed medical histories aid in pinpointing the root cause.

- **Autoimmune Disorders:** Given the autoimmune nature of Addison's Disease, distinguishing it from other autoimmune conditions, such as rheumatoid arthritis or systemic lupus erythematosus, is crucial. Specific autoantibody testing helps in confirming the autoimmune etiology of Addison's.

The differential diagnosis of Addison's Disease involves a meticulous evaluation of symptoms, comprehensive laboratory testing, and imaging studies. Collaboration between healthcare professionals from various specialties is often required to rule out potential contributing factors. By systematically considering and eliminating other possible causes, clinicians can arrive at an accurate diagnosis and tailor appropriate management strategies for individuals presenting with symptoms suggestive of adrenal dysfunction.

# Chapter three

# Types of Addison's Disease

Addison's Disease encompasses primary and secondary forms. Primary Addison's results from autoimmune adrenalitis, where the body's immune system attacks and damages the adrenal glands. Secondary Addison's arises due to dysfunction in the pituitary or hypothalamus, leading to insufficient stimulation of cortisol production. Additionally, atypical forms may result from infections, tumors, or genetic factors. These variations highlight the diverse etiologies contributing to adrenal insufficiency, necessitating nuanced diagnostic approaches and tailored management strategies for each subtype.

## Primary vs. Secondary Addison's Disease

Addison's Disease, characterized by adrenal insufficiency, manifests in primary and secondary forms, each with distinct etiologies and underlying mechanisms.

## Primary Addison's Disease

**Autoimmune Adrenalitis:** Primary Addison's, also known as Addison's Disease proper, predominantly results from autoimmune adrenalitis. In this form, the body's immune system mistakenly identifies components of the adrenal glands, particularly the adrenal cortex, as foreign invaders and launches an autoimmune response. This autoimmune assault leads to chronic inflammation, gradual destruction of adrenal tissue, and compromised hormonal production. The specific trigger initiating this immune response remains elusive, but there is a notable association with genetic predispositions. The autoimmune nature is underscored by the presence of autoantibodies, particularly anti-21-hydroxylase antibodies, which target an enzyme crucial for cortisol synthesis.

**Gradual Onset and Progressive Nature:** Primary Addison's Disease often has an insidious onset, with symptoms manifesting gradually as the autoimmune process progresses. Fatigue, weight loss, hyperpigmentation, and electrolyte imbalances are characteristic features. The progressive decline in adrenal function results in chronic insufficiency, necessitating lifelong hormone replacement therapy to address cortisol and aldosterone deficiencies.

## Secondary Addison's Disease

**Pituitary or Hypothalamic Dysfunction:** Secondary Addison's Disease, distinct from the primary form, arises from dysfunction in the pituitary gland or hypothalamus, key components of the brain's endocrine control system. Tumors, infections, or structural issues affecting these regions can disrupt the production and release of adrenocorticotropic hormone (ACTH). ACTH, in turn, stimulates the adrenal glands to produce cortisol. In secondary Addison's, the insufficient ACTH stimulation leads to reduced cortisol synthesis despite structurally intact adrenal glands.

**Distinctive Hormonal Profile:** The hormonal deficiency in secondary Addison's Disease is primarily a consequence of impaired ACTH production. Unlike primary Addison's, there is no autoimmune destruction of the adrenal cortex. Consequently, mineralocorticoid function, regulated by aldosterone, may remain relatively intact, distinguishing secondary Addison's from the complete adrenal insufficiency observed in the primary form.

## Differential Diagnostic Features

**Diagnostic Challenges:** Distinguishing between primary and secondary Addison's Disease can pose diagnostic challenges due to overlapping symptoms. Both forms may present with fatigue, weight loss, and gastrointestinal disturbances. However, specific diagnostic markers, including cortisol and ACTH levels, help differentiate the two.

**Laboratory and Stimulation Tests:** Laboratory tests measuring basal cortisol and ACTH levels provide initial insights. In primary Addison's, cortisol levels are typically low, and ACTH levels are elevated due to the lack of negative feedback. In secondary Addison's, both cortisol and ACTH levels may be diminished. The cosyntropin stimulation test, assessing cortisol response to synthetic ACTH, aids in confirming adrenal function and distinguishing primary from secondary causes.

Understanding the distinctive features of primary and secondary Addison's Disease is pivotal for accurate diagnosis and tailored management. Primary Addison's, rooted in autoimmune processes, demands lifelong hormone replacement therapy. Secondary Addison's, often associated with underlying pituitary or hypothalamic dysfunction, requires addressing the specific hormonal deficiencies while considering the intact adrenal gland structure.

## Atypical Forms of Addison's Disease

While primary and secondary Addison's Disease represents the conventional manifestations, atypical forms introduce additional complexities to the landscape of adrenal insufficiency. These variations may arise from diverse etiologies, including infections, genetic factors, or unique clinical scenarios.

◆ **Infectious Etiologies:** Atypical forms of Addison's Disease can result from infections infiltrating the adrenal glands. Historically, tuberculosis was a prominent cause, causing inflammation and scarring that compromised adrenal function. Other infections, such as fungal infections (e.g., histoplasmosis, coccidioidomycosis), can similarly affect the adrenals, although these instances are relatively rare.

◆ **Genetic Factors:** Genetic predispositions can contribute to atypical forms, with certain familial patterns identified in adrenal insufficiency. Specific genetic markers, including those associated with the Human Leukocyte Antigen (HLA) system, have been linked to susceptibility. Familial forms may present with unique characteristics, emphasizing the role of genetic factors in shaping an individual's vulnerability.

◆ **Adrenal Hemorrhage:** Atypical Addison's Disease may result from adrenal hemorrhage, particularly in scenarios involving trauma, infections, or complications during childbirth. Neonatal adrenal hemorrhage, occurring in newborns, is a distinct entity contributing to adrenal insufficiency and requires specialized consideration.

◆ **Medication-Induced Addison's:** Certain medications, especially long-term use of glucocorticoids like prednisone, can induce adrenal insufficiency. Abrupt cessation of these medications can lead to adrenal crisis, emphasizing the importance of careful management to prevent complications. Surgical removal of adrenal glands for conditions like tumors or cancer can also result in Addison's Disease, requiring strategic hormonal replacement therapy.

◆ **Idiopathic Addison's Disease:** In a subset of cases, Addison's Disease may lack a clear identifiable cause, leading to its classification as idiopathic adrenal insufficiency. The term "idiopathic" is applied when the etiology remains elusive despite thorough investigation. This atypical variant underscores the gaps in current knowledge and highlights the ongoing need for research to unravel the complexities of adrenal dysfunction.

Atypical forms of Addison's Disease present unique diagnostic and management challenges, requiring a nuanced approach tailored to the specific underlying causes. The diversity of etiologies emphasizes the intricate nature of adrenal insufficiency and the continuous exploration needed to comprehensively understand and address these atypical manifestations.

# Chapter four

# Treatment Options for

# Addison's Disease

The cornerstone of Addison's Disease management involves lifelong hormone replacement therapy to address cortisol and aldosterone deficiencies. Glucocorticoid medications, such as hydrocortisone or prednisone, mimic cortisol's effects, managing symptoms and supporting metabolism. Mineralocorticoid replacement, often with fludrocortisone, helps regulate electrolyte balance. Individualized dosing is crucial, and adjustments may be needed during periods of stress. Patient education on medication management, stress response, and the recognition of adrenal crisis is integral for effective treatment. Regular medical monitoring ensures optimal hormone replacement, promoting a balanced and healthy life for individuals with Addison's Disease.

# Hormone Replacement Therapy in Addison's Disease

Hormone replacement therapy (HRT) forms the bedrock of managing Addison's Disease, aiming to compensate for deficient cortisol and aldosterone production. Tailored administration of glucocorticoids and mineralocorticoids is essential, reflecting the nuanced nature of adrenal insufficiency.

## Glucocorticoid Replacement

Hydrocortisone or Prednisone: Mimicking the body's natural cortisol rhythm is crucial. Hydrocortisone, often preferred for its short duration of action, closely replicates the circadian cortisol pattern. Prednisone, with a longer duration, may be used but requires careful dose adjustments.

**Mineralocorticoid Replacement:**
Fludrocortisone: Addressing aldosterone deficiency, fludrocortisone helps regulate sodium and potassium balance. Adjustments in fludrocortisone dosage are guided by monitoring blood pressure, electrolyte levels, and clinical symptoms.

**Things to note;**

**Individualized Dosing and Stress Response:**
Dosages are tailored to individual needs, reflecting factors such as age, weight, activity levels, and stress. Increased doses during illness, surgery, or stressful situations are often necessary to meet heightened cortisol demands. Close monitoring and prompt adjustments prevent adrenal crisis during such periods.

**Balancing Act:**
Achieving a delicate equilibrium in hormone replacement is an ongoing challenge. Overreplacement risks complications such as osteoporosis and hypertension, while underreplacement leads to symptoms of adrenal insufficiency. Close collaboration between patients and healthcare providers is imperative

for fine-tuning HRT regimens, ensuring optimal quality of life for those with Addison's Disease.

In summary, hormone replacement therapy in Addison's Disease is a dynamic and personalized endeavor. Tailoring glucocorticoid and mineralocorticoid replacement, emphasizing patient education, and maintaining vigilant monitoring constitute the pillars of effective management, empowering individuals to lead healthy and balanced lives despite adrenal insufficiency.

# Medications in Addison's Disease

## Corticosteroids

**Hydrocortisone (Cortisol):** The preferred glucocorticoid for replacement therapy, hydrocortisone closely mimics the body's natural cortisol rhythm. Its short duration of action allows for dose adjustments to match physiological needs, including stress responses. Splitting the daily dose ensures a diurnal cortisol pattern, aligning with the body's natural circadian rhythm.

**Prednisone:** A longer-acting glucocorticoid, prednisone is an alternative to hydrocortisone. Its extended duration requires careful dosing adjustments. It is often chosen when once-daily dosing is preferred, but vigilant monitoring is necessary to avoid over-replacement.

**Dexamethasone:** Infrequently used due to its prolonged action and potential for adrenal suppression, dexamethasone may be employed in specific situations. It requires cautious dosing and monitoring, particularly in avoiding excessive suppression of the hypothalamic-pituitary-adrenal (HPA) axis.

## Mineralocorticoids

**Fludrocortisone**: Addressing aldosterone deficiency, fludrocortisone is the primary mineralocorticoid used in Addison's Disease. Its pharmacological profile aids in regulating sodium and potassium balance, thereby maintaining blood pressure and preventing electrolyte imbalances. Dosing adjustments are guided by blood pressure, electrolyte levels, and clinical symptoms.

In conclusion, medications, particularly corticosteroids and mineralocorticoids, play a pivotal role in treating Addison's Disease.

# Individualized Treatment Plans in Addison's Disease

The management of Addison's Disease hinges on individualized treatment plans, recognizing the nuanced nature of adrenal insufficiency. Each patient's unique characteristics, lifestyle, and stress responses demand personalized approaches to hormone replacement therapy (HRT).

**Customized Hormone Replacement**
Glucocorticoid (e.g., hydrocortisone, prednisone) and mineralocorticoid (fludrocortisone) dosages are tailored to individual needs, accounting for factors like age, weight, and activity levels. Balancing cortisol rhythms and maintaining electrolyte equilibrium are paramount.

**Stress Dosing Principles**
Educating patients on stress dosing is fundamental. Recognizing situations that demand

increased glucocorticoid doses, such as illness or surgery, empowers individuals to prevent adrenal crisis during stressors.

## Regular Monitoring

Routine blood tests, including cortisol and electrolyte panels, ensure ongoing optimization. Monitoring provides insights into the effectiveness of treatment, guiding adjustments to prevent under-replacement or over-replacement complications.

## Lifestyle Considerations

Lifestyle factors, including diet, exercise, and stress management, are integral components. Recognizing how these elements influence hormonal needs aids in refining treatment plans for sustained well-being.

## Patient Education and Empowerment

Patient education is central to adherence and successful management. Understanding symptoms, stress dosing, and the importance of regular follow-ups empowers individuals to actively participate in their care.

## Collaborative Care

Collaborative relationships between patients and healthcare providers, particularly endocrinologists, foster ongoing communication and support. Regular follow-up appointments allow for adjustments and address evolving needs. By embracing an individualized treatment paradigm, healthcare providers ensure that individuals with Addison's Disease receive care attuned to their unique physiology and circumstances, fostering not only symptom control but also an enhanced quality of life.

# Chapter five

# Managing Daily Life with

# Addison's Disease

Daily life with Addison's Disease involves vigilant self-care to maintain hormonal equilibrium. Adherence to prescribed medication regimens, including glucocorticoids and mineralocorticoids, is paramount. Understanding stress dosing principles empowers individuals to navigate illness or other stressors safely. Regular monitoring through blood tests ensures optimal hormone replacement. Lifestyle considerations, from diet to stress management, play pivotal roles. Educating oneself on symptoms and proactive engagement with healthcare providers fosters a collaborative approach. By embracing these strategies, individuals with Addison's Disease can effectively manage daily challenges and lead fulfilling lives.

# Lifestyle Adjustments for Well-being in Addison's Disease

Living with Addison's Disease necessitates thoughtful lifestyle adjustments to promote overall health and mitigate the impact of adrenal insufficiency. Key considerations include:

**Diet and Nutrition in Addison's Disease**
Maintaining a well balanced is pivotal for individuals with Addison's Disease, addressing specific needs associated with adrenal insufficiency. Dietary considerations play a crucial role in supporting overall health and compensating for deficiencies in cortisol and aldosterone. Key aspects include:

✓ **Sodium Intake:** Adequate sodium is essential to counteract the sodium loss resulting from aldosterone deficiency. Individuals are often advised to slightly increase their salt intake, especially during warmer weather or periods of increased physical activity. This helps prevent dehydration and electrolyte imbalances.

✓ **Balanced Nutrition:** Ensuring a diet rich in essential nutrients supports sustained energy levels and overall well-being. A balanced intake of proteins, carbohydrates, healthy fats, vitamins, and minerals contributes to optimal nutrition.

✓ **Hydration:** Proper hydration is paramount. Individuals with Addison's Disease may be prone to dehydration due to salt-wasting. Maintaining adequate fluid intake helps prevent electrolyte imbalances and supports cardiovascular health.

✓ **Timing of Meals:** Consistent meal timing is beneficial for managing blood sugar levels and cortisol rhythms. Regular, well-timed meals contribute to stable energy levels and help avoid hypoglycemia.

✓ **Cortisol-Friendly Snacks:** Incorporating cortisol-friendly snacks between meals can help stabilize blood sugar levels. Nutrient-dense options, such as nuts, fruits, or yogurt, provide sustained energy without causing rapid blood sugar fluctuations.

✓ **Adaptation to Stressors:** During periods of illness or stress, adjustments in diet may be necessary. Increased fluid intake, easy-to-digest foods, and adherence to stress dosing principles ensure adequate support for cortisol demands.

✓ **Monitoring Blood Sugar:** Individuals with Addison's Disease should monitor their blood sugar levels, especially when adjusting medication doses or during illness. Maintaining stable blood sugar levels is crucial for preventing hypoglycemia, a common concern in adrenal insufficiency.

✓ **Collaboration with Healthcare Providers:** collaboration with healthcare providers, including dietitians or nutritionists, is beneficial for tailoring dietary recommendations to individual needs. Regular monitoring of nutritional status ensures comprehensive care.

By embracing these dietary principles, individuals with Addison's Disease can optimize their nutritional intake, support hormonal balance, and enhance overall health. Thoughtful dietary choices, coupled with ongoing collaboration with healthcare professionals, contribute to a holistic approach to managing the complexities of adrenal insufficiency.

# Exercise and Physical Activity in Addison's Disease:

Engaging in regular exercise is a cornerstone of a healthy lifestyle, even for individuals with Addison's Disease. However, due to the unique considerations associated with adrenal insufficiency, thoughtful planning and adjustments are necessary to ensure safe and beneficial physical activity.

✓ **Moderate and Consistent Exercise:** Moderate and consistent exercise is generally well-tolerated and can contribute to overall well-being. Activities such as brisk walking, swimming, or cycling can enhance cardiovascular health without excessive stress on the adrenal glands.

✓ **Stress Dosing for Intense Workouts:** For more intense workouts or strenuous physical activities, individuals may need to implement stress dosing principles. Increasing glucocorticoid doses before, during, and after such activities helps meet heightened cortisol demands, preventing adrenal crisis.

✓ **Hydration and Electrolyte Balance:** Adequate hydration is crucial during exercise to prevent dehydration and maintain electrolyte balance. Individuals with Addison's Disease should pay attention to fluid intake, particularly in warm weather, to offset potential salt-wasting.

✓ **Monitoring and Adjustments:** Regular monitoring of symptoms, including fatigue, dizziness, or weakness, is essential during and after exercise. Adjustments in medication doses or timing may be needed based on individual responses to physical activity.

✓ **Adapting to Stressful Situations:** Stressful situations, whether physical or emotional, demand a proactive approach. Understanding how stress impacts cortisol needs and adjusting medication accordingly helps individuals navigate such scenarios without compromising well-being.

✓ **Individualized Approach:** Recognizing that each person's tolerance for exercise varies, an individualized approach is crucial. Factors such as age, fitness level, and overall health should be considered when developing an exercise routine.

✓ **Collaborative Care:** Collaboration with healthcare providers, including input from endocrinologists or exercise physiologists, ensures that exercise plans align with an individual's specific needs and medical considerations. Regular check-ins and adjustments contribute to a holistic approach to well-being.

By incorporating exercise into their routine, individuals with Addison's Disease can enjoy the physical and mental health benefits associated with an active lifestyle. Thoughtful planning, adherence to stress dosing principles, and ongoing collaboration with healthcare professionals empower individuals to strike a balance between physical activity and adrenal health, fostering a fulfilling and active life.

## Other important lifestyle adjustments

**Stress Management:** Incorporating stress-reducing practices, such as mindfulness, meditation, or yoga, aids in managing cortisol responses. Stress can exacerbate symptoms, and proactive stress management is integral to overall well-being.

**Sleep Hygiene:** Ensuring sufficient and quality sleep supports adrenal health and contributes to overall vitality. Establishing a consistent sleep routine helps maintain circadian rhythms.

**Medication Adherence:** Strict adherence to prescribed medication regimens, including glucocorticoids and mineralocorticoids, is fundamental. Consistent dosing, especially during stressful situations, prevents adrenal crises and sustains hormonal balance.

**Temperature Regulation:** Individuals should be mindful of temperature extremes. Hot weather can increase the risk of dehydration, requiring adjustments in fluid intake, while cold weather may demand additional stress dosing.

**Regular Monitoring and Healthcare Engagement:** Regular medical check-ups, including blood tests, are crucial for monitoring hormone levels and adjusting medication as needed. Ongoing communication with healthcare providers fosters a proactive and collaborative approach to care.

**Emergency Preparedness:** Creating an emergency plan, including educating family members or close contacts about the condition and necessary interventions during adrenal crises, is essential. Carrying an emergency kit with injectable cortisol is often recommended.

By integrating these lifestyle adjustments, individuals with Addison's Disease can enhance their daily well-being and effectively navigate the complexities associated with adrenal insufficiency. Thoughtful choices, proactive self-care, and ongoing collaboration with healthcare providers contribute to a balanced and fulfilling life despite the challenges posed by the condition.

# Chapter six

# Complications and Associated Conditions in Addison's Disease

Addison's Disease, while primarily characterized by adrenal insufficiency, can give rise to complications and associated conditions. Notable complications include adrenal crisis, a life-threatening emergency marked by severe hypotension and electrolyte imbalances. Osteoporosis may develop due to prolonged cortisol deficiency. Associated autoimmune disorders, such as thyroid dysfunction or diabetes, may coexist. Vigilant monitoring, adherence to treatment regimens, and proactive management of complications are integral aspects of care, ensuring individuals with Addison's Disease navigate the complexities and maintain optimal health. Regular medical check-ups are essential for comprehensive evaluation and early intervention if complications arise.

# Adrenal Crisis in Addison's Disease

Adrenal crisis represents a severe and potentially life-threatening complication of Addison's Disease, demanding swift recognition and immediate intervention. This crisis arises from a profound deficiency in cortisol, the crucial hormone produced by the adrenal glands. Several triggers can precipitate an adrenal crisis, including illness, trauma, surgery, or inadequate hormone replacement therapy.

**Symptoms and Signs**
The onset of an adrenal crisis is marked by symptoms such as extreme fatigue, weakness, dizziness, nausea, vomiting, and abdominal pain. Individuals may experience confusion, low blood pressure, and dehydration. In severe cases, loss of consciousness can occur.

## Risk Factors

Individuals with Addison's Disease are particularly vulnerable to adrenal crises, and certain factors increase the risk. Skipping medication doses, sudden withdrawal from corticosteroid therapy, or failure to adjust doses during stress or illness can precipitate a crisis.

## Emergency Intervention

Immediate medical attention is paramount. Emergency measures include administering intravenous fluids to address dehydration, and intravenous or intramuscular corticosteroids to rapidly replenish cortisol levels. These interventions stabilize blood pressure and reverse the cascade of symptoms associated with adrenal crisis.

## Prevention and Preparedness

Preventing adrenal crises involves diligent management of Addison's Disease. Adherence to prescribed medication regimens, especially during times of illness or stress, is crucial. Patients and caregivers should be educated on recognizing early signs of crisis and implementing stress dosing principles promptly.

## Emergency Kit

Many individuals with Addison's Disease carry emergency kits containing injectable hydrocortisone for self-administration during crises. This immediate intervention can be vital while awaiting professional medical assistance.

**Medical Follow-up**

After an adrenal crisis, close medical follow-up is essential. The circumstances leading to the crisis are assessed, and adjustments to medication regimens or additional precautions may be implemented to prevent recurrence.

Recognizing the gravity of adrenal crises and adopting proactive measures are central to the management of Addison's Disease.

# Autoimmune Disorders in the Context of Addison's Disease

Addison's Disease is predominantly rooted in autoimmune adrenalitis, underscoring the intricate relationship between adrenal insufficiency and autoimmune disorders. Autoimmune mechanisms involve the body's immune system mistakenly attacking its tissues, in this case, the adrenal glands. However, the autoimmune association extends beyond the adrenal cortex to encompass a spectrum of related conditions.

**Polyglandular Autoimmune Syndromes (PAS)**
Addison's Disease is frequently part of broader polyglandular autoimmune syndromes, such as APS-1 and APS-2. These syndromes involve autoimmune dysfunction affecting multiple endocrine glands. APS-1 is characterized by diverse autoimmune manifestations, including Addison's, autoimmune thyroiditis, and mucocutaneous candidiasis.

**Autoimmune Thyroid Disorders**
The co-occurrence of Addison's Disease with autoimmune thyroid disorders, such as Hashimoto's thyroiditis or Graves' disease, is common. Shared autoimmune mechanisms contribute to the simultaneous dysfunction of the adrenal glands and thyroid.

**Type 1 Diabetes Mellitus:**
Type 1 diabetes, another autoimmune condition, may coexist with Addison's Disease. Both conditions involve the immune system targeting specific tissues—the pancreatic beta cells in diabetes and the adrenal cortex in Addison's.

**Rheumatological Autoimmune Disorders**
Rheumatoid arthritis, systemic lupus erythematosus, and other rheumatological autoimmune disorders can present alongside Addison's Disease. Shared autoimmune predispositions contribute to the clustering of these conditions in certain individuals.

**Autoimmune Polyendocrine Syndrome (APS)**
APS encompasses a spectrum of autoimmune disorders affecting multiple endocrine organs. APS-2 is particularly relevant to Addison's Disease, commonly involving autoimmune adrenalitis alongside thyroid and pancreatic dysfunction. Understanding the broader landscape of autoimmune disorders associated with Addison's Disease enhances clinical insight, prompting thorough evaluations and comprehensive care.

## Mental Health Considerations in Addison's Disease

Managing Addison's Disease extends beyond the physical realm, with crucial implications for mental health. The chronic nature of the condition, potential complications, and the need for lifelong medication adherence can impact emotional well-being.

✓ **Coping with Chronicity:** The chronic nature of Addison's Disease requires ongoing management, which may lead to emotional challenges. Individuals may navigate feelings of frustration, anxiety, or uncertainty regarding their health.

✓ **Impact of Symptoms:** Symptomatic manifestations, especially fatigue and weakness, can affect daily life and mood. Coping strategies and adaptive approaches become essential in maintaining a positive mental outlook.

✓ **Medication Impact:** Corticosteroid medications, while vital for hormone replacement, can influence mood and mental health. Individuals may experience mood swings, anxiety, or insomnia, necessitating open communication with healthcare providers for adjustments.

✓ **Stress Management:** Stress, whether physical or emotional, plays a significant role in adrenal function. Adopting stress management techniques, such as mindfulness, meditation, or counseling, contributes to mental resilience and overall well-being.

✓ **Social Support:** Building a robust support network, including friends, family, and healthcare providers, fosters emotional resilience. Open communication about the challenges of living with Addison's Disease facilitates understanding and empathy.

**Routine Mental Health Check-ins**
Incorporating routine mental health check-ins as part of overall care ensures holistic support. Healthcare providers, including mental health professionals, play a vital role in addressing emotional concerns and offering tailored interventions.

Balancing the physical and mental aspects of Addison's Disease is essential for comprehensive well-being. Recognizing the interconnectedness of physical symptoms and emotional health, individuals can cultivate resilience, seek timely support, and foster a positive mindset to navigate the complexities of living with a chronic endocrine condition.

# Chapter seven

# Medical Monitoring in

# Addison's Disease

Regular medical monitoring is a cornerstone of managing Addison's Disease, ensuring optimal hormone replacement and early detection of potential complications. Blood tests, including cortisol and electrolyte panels, provide insights into hormonal levels. Monitoring helps healthcare providers tailor medication regimens, preventing under-replacement or over-replacement. Periodic check-ups allow for a comprehensive evaluation of overall health and adjustments to treatment plans. This vigilant approach empowers individuals to proactively manage their condition, fostering long-term well-being and minimizing the risk of adrenal crises or associated complications.

The Significance of Regular Check-ups in Addison's Disease Management

Regular check-ups are indispensable in the comprehensive management of Addison's Disease, ensuring ongoing health, medication optimization, and early intervention when needed. These appointments serve multiple crucial purposes.

- **Hormone Level Monitoring:** Regular blood tests, including cortisol and electrolyte panels, enable healthcare providers to monitor hormone levels. This aids in assessing the effectiveness of hormone replacement therapy and detecting any imbalances that may arise.

- **Medication Adjustments:** Check-ups provide opportunities for healthcare providers to adjust medication dosages based on individual responses, ensuring that hormone replacement remains tailored to each patient's needs. This dynamic approach minimizes the risk of under-replacement or over-replacement.

- **Symptom Evaluation:** Evaluation of symptoms, both physical and emotional, allows healthcare providers to gauge the impact of Addison's Disease on an individual's daily life. Addressing emerging symptoms promptly enhances overall well-being.

- **Complication Prevention:** Regular check-ups facilitate the early detection and prevention of potential complications associated with Addison's Disease. From addressing adrenal crises to managing coexisting autoimmune conditions, proactive measures can be taken to mitigate risks.

- **Psychosocial Support:** Check-ups provide opportunities for healthcare providers to assess psychosocial aspects of well-being. Addressing emotional challenges, offering support, and connecting individuals with mental health resources contribute to holistic care.

- **Patient Education:** Regular appointments serve as valuable opportunities for patient education. Individuals receive updated information on the latest advancements in Addison's management, reinforcing the importance of adherence to treatment plans and stress dosing principles.

In summary, regular check-ups are a linchpin in the ongoing care of individuals with Addison's

Disease. These appointments offer a comprehensive view of an individual's health, allowing for tailored interventions, preventive measures, and continuous support.

## Blood Tests and Monitoring Parameters in Addison's Disease

In the management of Addison's Disease, blood tests and monitoring parameters play a pivotal role in assessing hormonal balance, guiding treatment adjustments, and detecting potential complications. Key aspects of this monitoring approach include:

**Cortisol Levels:** Regular measurement of cortisol levels is fundamental. Blood tests, often taken in the morning to align with the body's natural cortisol peak, provide insights into the adequacy of glucocorticoid replacement. Monitoring cortisol helps prevent under-replacement, ensuring optimal symptom control.

**Electrolyte Panels:** Monitoring electrolyte levels, including sodium and potassium, is crucial in addressing mineralocorticoid deficiencies.

Electrolyte imbalances can lead to complications such as dehydration and cardiovascular issues. Regular panels guide adjustments in mineralocorticoid replacement, promoting overall health.

**Blood Pressure**: Blood pressure monitoring is integral, especially in individuals receiving mineralocorticoid replacement. Maintaining appropriate blood pressure levels helps prevent complications related to aldosterone deficiency, such as hypotension.

**Blood Sugar Levels:** Individuals with Addison's Disease, particularly those with coexisting diabetes, benefit from monitoring blood sugar levels. Corticosteroid medications can influence glucose metabolism, and regular checks assist in managing diabetes effectively.

**Lipid Profiles:** Corticosteroid therapy may impact lipid metabolism, influencing cholesterol levels. Periodic lipid profiles contribute to cardiovascular risk assessment and guide lifestyle and, if needed, pharmacological interventions.

**Renal Function Tests:** Considering the role of aldosterone in renal function, regular monitoring of kidney function is essential. Assessing parameters like creatinine and blood urea nitrogen helps detect potential renal complications.

**Comprehensive Metabolic Panels:** Comprehensive metabolic panels provide a holistic overview of an individual's metabolic health. Monitoring liver function, kidney function, and electrolyte balance ensures a thorough assessment of overall well-being.

**Patient Feedback and Symptoms:** Equally important is gathering subjective feedback from patients about their symptoms and well-being. Patient-reported experiences guide healthcare providers in understanding the impact of Addison's Disease on daily life, informing targeted interventions.

Regular blood tests and monitoring parameters enable a proactive and individualized approach to Addison's Disease management. This dynamic monitoring strategy ensures that hormone replacement therapy remains tailored to each individual's needs, fostering optimal health and minimizing the risk of complications associated with adrenal insufficiency.

# Emergency Preparedness in Addison's Disease

Emergency preparedness is paramount for individuals with Addison's Disease, offering a proactive approach to handle potential adrenal crises. Key elements of preparedness include

✧ **Education and Awareness:** Thorough education on recognizing early signs and symptoms of adrenal crisis empowers individuals to act swiftly. Understanding the importance of stress dosing principles during illness or stress is central to emergency readiness.

✧ **Emergency Kit:** Carrying an emergency kit containing injectable hydrocortisone is a crucial aspect of preparedness. This immediate intervention can be vital while awaiting professional medical assistance, especially in situations where oral medications may be challenging.

✧ **Communication and Alerting Others:** Informing close contacts, family members, and colleagues about Addison's Disease and its potential emergencies ensures a support network is aware of necessary interventions. Clear communication aids in a timely response.

✧ **Emergency Action Plan:** Developing and regularly reviewing an emergency action plan with healthcare providers helps outline specific steps to take during adrenal crises. This plan may include instructions for self-administering medication, seeking immediate medical attention, and contacting healthcare providers.

✧ **Recognition of Triggers:** Identifying triggers that may lead to adrenal crises, such as illness, surgery, or extreme stress, allows for anticipatory measures. Stress management techniques and preventive stress dosing during known stressors contribute to crisis prevention.

✧ **Regular Follow-up:** Regular medical check-ups ensure ongoing evaluation of Addison's management. Healthcare providers can assess emergency preparedness, adjust treatment plans, and address any emerging concerns.

By fostering a culture of preparedness, individuals with Addison's Disease can navigate potential emergencies with confidence. Education, well-defined action plans, and effective communication serve as pillars of emergency readiness, contributing to a proactive and empowered approach in managing adrenal insufficiency.

# Chapter eight

# Support Systems in Addison's

# Disease

Building a robust support system is indispensable for individuals with Addison's Disease. Family, friends, and healthcare providers form the pillars of emotional and practical assistance. Understanding the complexities of adrenal insufficiency, these support networks offer empathy, encouragement, and, when needed, help in emergencies. Open communication fosters collaboration in managing the condition, enhancing overall resilience and well-being for those navigating the challenges of living with Addison's.

# Support Groups and Communities in Addison's Disease

Engaging with support groups and communities proves invaluable for individuals navigating the complexities of Addison's Disease. These communities offer a unique space for shared experiences, empathy, and practical insights. Key aspects of the support garnered from these groups include:

✧ **Shared Understanding:** Connecting with others facing similar challenges fosters a deep sense of understanding. Shared experiences create a supportive environment where individuals can express concerns, share coping strategies, and find solace in the common journey of living with adrenal insufficiency.

✧ **Emotional Support:** Emotional well-being is nurtured through the empathy and encouragement provided within these communities. Whether individuals are newly diagnosed or managing the condition for years, the emotional support gained from shared narratives contributes to a sense of community and belonging.

✧ **Practical Tips and Advice:** Practical insights and advice on managing daily life with Addison's Disease are often shared within these communities. Tips on medication management, stress coping strategies, and navigating healthcare systems provide valuable guidance for individuals seeking to optimize their well-being.

✧ **Education and Awareness:** Support groups serve as platforms for education and awareness. Members exchange information on the latest medical advancements, treatment options, and lifestyle adjustments. This collective knowledge empowers individuals to make informed decisions about their health.

✧ **Online Platforms and Local Meetings:** Online forums, social media groups, and local support group meetings offer various avenues for connection. Virtual spaces enable individuals worldwide to participate, while local meetings provide opportunities for face-to-face interactions and community building.

✧ **Advocacy and Empowerment:** Support communities often engage in advocacy efforts, promoting awareness about Addison's Disease and advocating for better understanding within the broader community. This collective empowerment contributes to the destigmatization of the condition and fosters a sense of resilience.

✧ **Encouragement in Adversity:** During challenging times, such as adrenal crises or setbacks in managing the condition, the encouragement and shared wisdom from fellow community members become invaluable. This network serves as a safety net, offering encouragement and practical guidance during times of adversity.

Engaging with support groups and communities in Addison's Disease is not just about shared struggles; it is a celebration of shared victories, resilience, and collective empowerment. The connections forged within these groups contribute significantly to the overall well-being and quality of life for individuals navigating the journey of adrenal insufficiency.

# Psychological Support in Addison's Disease

Living with Addison's Disease necessitates a holistic approach that extends beyond physical health, acknowledging the profound impact on mental well-being. Psychological support plays a pivotal role in fostering mental resilience

- ✧ **Coping with Chronicity:** Managing a chronic condition like Addison's Disease requires coping strategies for the emotional toll it may take. Psychological support provides a space to explore and implement effective coping mechanisms.

- ✧ **Emotional Impact of Symptoms:** Symptoms such as fatigue and weakness can have significant emotional ramifications. Psychological support helps individuals navigate and understand the emotional impact of these symptoms, fostering emotional resilience.

- ✧ **Medication-Related Challenges:** Corticosteroid medications, integral to Addison's treatment, can influence mood and mental health. Psychological support assists individuals in addressing and adapting to any challenges related to medication effects on emotions and mental well-being.

✧ **Stress Management:** The role of stress in adrenal function makes stress management crucial. Psychological support equips individuals with effective stress management techniques, promoting emotional balance and minimizing the impact of stressors.

✧ **Education and Empowerment:** Understanding the psychological aspects of living with Addison's is empowering. Psychological support provides education on the interconnectedness of mental and physical health, fostering a holistic approach to well-being.

✧ **Addressing Anxiety and Uncertainty:**Anxiety and uncertainty about the future are common emotional responses to chronic illness. Psychological support offers tools and strategies to address these concerns, promoting a sense of control and empowerment.

✧ **Stigma Reduction:** Supportive environments contribute to destigmatizing Addison's

Disease. Psychological support helps individuals navigate societal perceptions, fostering a positive self-image and reducing the emotional impact of potential stigmatization.

By addressing the psychological dimensions of living with Addison's Disease, individuals can cultivate mental resilience, navigate emotional challenges, and foster a positive mindset.

## Educating Family and Friends about Addison's Disease

Educating family and friends about Addison's Disease is paramount to fostering a supportive environment. Providing information on the condition, its management, and potential challenges ensures a foundation of understanding. Emphasizing the importance of medication adherence, stress dosing principles, and recognizing signs of adrenal crisis equips loved ones to offer informed assistance. By sharing insights into lifestyle adjustments and emotional aspects, individuals with Addison's cultivate a network of understanding, enabling their close circles to provide empathetic support and participate actively in the journey of managing this chronic endocrine condition.

# Chapter nine

# Research and Future Developments in Addison's Disease

Ongoing research in Addison's Disease focuses on refining treatment approaches, understanding genetic predispositions, and exploring potential biomarkers for early detection. Advances aim to enhance hormone replacement therapies, minimize side effects, and improve overall patient outcomes. As science progresses, these developments hold promise for a more nuanced and personalized approach to managing Addison's Disease, offering hope for increased effectiveness and improved quality of life for those affected by this endocrine disorder.

## Current Research in Addison's Disease

Contemporary research in Addison's Disease is marked by a multifaceted exploration of underlying mechanisms, novel treatment modalities, and refined diagnostic tools.
**Key areas of focus include:**

- **Genetic Insights:**Unraveling the genetic basis of Addison's Disease remains a priority. Researchers are identifying specific genetic markers associated with increased susceptibility, shedding light on the intricate interplay of genetics in adrenal insufficiency.

- **Precision Medicine Approaches:** Efforts to move towards precision medicine in Addison's involve tailoring treatments based on individual genetic and molecular profiles. This approach aims to optimize hormone replacement therapy, minimizing side effects and improving overall therapeutic outcomes.

- **Biomarkers for Early Detection:** Identification of reliable biomarkers for early detection of adrenal dysfunction is a key avenue of research. Biomarkers could enable timely intervention and potentially prevent the progression of the disease, enhancing overall prognoses.

- **Immunomodulation Strategies:** Given the autoimmune nature of Addison's, exploring immunomodulation strategies is underway. Researchers are investigating ways to modulate the immune response, potentially halting or slowing down the autoimmune destruction of adrenal tissue.

- **Long-Term Treatment Effects:** Research delves into the long-term effects of corticosteroid therapy, seeking to minimize side effects associated with extended medication use. Balancing effective hormone replacement with mitigating potential complications is a critical focus.

- **Patient-Reported Outcomes:** Understanding the impact of Addison's on patients' lives involves research on patient-reported outcomes. Exploring the physical, emotional, and social aspects of living with adrenal insufficiency provides valuable insights for comprehensive care.

- **Technological Innovations:** Advancements in technology contribute to monitoring and managing Addison's Disease. Wearable devices and telemedicine solutions are being explored to enhance remote patient monitoring, improving accessibility to healthcare for individuals with Addison's.

As research in Addison's Disease evolves, the collective efforts of scientists, clinicians, and patient communities contribute to a deeper understanding of the condition. The goal is to translate these insights into more effective, personalized, and patient-centric approaches to managing adrenal insufficiency.

## Potential Breakthroughs in Addison's Disease

Anticipated breakthroughs in Addison's Disease research hold the promise of transforming management strategies and improving overall outcomes for individuals with adrenal insufficiency. Several areas exhibit potential for groundbreaking advancements:

✓ **Immunomodulation Therapies:** Innovations in immunomodulation therapies aim to modulate the immune response responsible for autoimmune destruction of the adrenal glands. This breakthrough could potentially halt or slow the progression of Addison's Disease, offering a disease-modifying approach.

✓ **Stem Cell Therapies:** Exploration of stem cell therapies holds significant promise. Researchers are investigating the potential of regenerating damaged adrenal tissue using stem cells, presenting a revolutionary avenue for restoring proper adrenal function.

✓ **Precision Medicine and Personalized Treatments:** Advancements in precision medicine aim to tailor treatments based on individual genetic and molecular profiles. This personalized approach could optimize hormone replacement therapy, minimize side effects, and enhance the overall effectiveness of treatment regimens.

✓ **Gene Therapy:** Gene therapy research seeks to address the root genetic causes of Addison's Disease. Pioneering approaches may involve introducing corrected genes to prevent or counteract the autoimmune attack on the adrenal glands.

✓ **Biomarkers for Early Detection:** Identifying reliable biomarkers for early detection is a crucial area of investigation. Breakthroughs in this realm could revolutionize diagnosis, enabling timely intervention before significant adrenal damage occurs.

✓ **Advanced Monitoring Technologies:** Integration of advanced monitoring technologies, such as wearable devices and continuous glucose monitoring, is poised to enhance real-time tracking of cortisol levels. These breakthroughs may empower individuals with Addison's to proactively manage their condition and optimize treatment plans.

✓ **Multidisciplinary Care Models:** Future breakthroughs may involve the development of comprehensive multidisciplinary care models. Integrating various medical specialties, including endocrinology, genetics, and immunology, could result in holistic approaches to managing Addison's Disease.

While these potential breakthroughs represent exciting prospects, it's essential to approach them with cautious optimism, recognizing the complexities of translating research findings into practical and safe clinical applications.

# Chapter 10

# Personal Stories and

# Perspectives

Beyond medical literature and research, the narratives of individuals living with Addison's Disease provide invaluable insights into the challenges, triumphs, and resilience inherent in managing this endocrine disorder. Personal stories and perspectives contribute significantly to the broader understanding of Addison's in several ways

✓ **Emotional Connection:** Personal stories forge emotional connections, allowing others to empathize with the unique journeys of those navigating adrenal insufficiency. Sharing experiences fosters a sense of community and understanding among individuals with Addison's and their support networks.

✓ **Real-World Challenges:** These narratives shed light on the day-to-day challenges faced by individuals with Addison's, from medication management to coping with symptoms. Real-world perspectives provide practical insights that complement clinical knowledge, offering a more holistic view of the condition.

✓ **Coping Strategies:** Personal stories often illuminate effective coping strategies employed by individuals with Addison's. Whether it's navigating work-life balance, handling stress, or addressing emotional well-being, these insights offer a reservoir of wisdom for others facing similar circumstances.

✓ **Treatment Adaptations:** Understanding how individuals adapt their treatment regimens to suit their lifestyles is crucial. Personal stories provide examples of successful treatment adaptations, highlighting the importance of individualized approaches to managing adrenal insufficiency.

✓ **Advocacy and Awareness:** Personal narratives serve as powerful advocacy tools, raising awareness about Addison's Disease within the broader community. By sharing their stories, individuals become advocates for increased understanding, reducing stigma, and fostering a supportive environment.

✓ **Resilience and Triumphs:** Personal stories underscore the resilience of individuals with Addison's. Narratives of triumph over adversity, successful management strategies, and achieving life goals inspire others facing similar challenges, offering hope and encouragement.

✓ **Educational Value:** Personal stories contribute to the educational landscape of Addison's Disease. Whether shared through blogs, social media, or patient support groups, these narratives provide a wealth of experiential knowledge that complements clinical information.

## True life story from a patient

I am 42 years old, I live in Texas USA. I grappled with an invisible illness that went unnoticed by my family and doctor. My children, aged 12 and 9, were my daily challenge as I struggled to maintain the household.

The first sign of my ailment, were darkening of my skin and weight loss, which was dismissed by my family doctor .

As time passed, my health deteriorated. My blood pressure started get so low. I had an irresistible craving for pizza and other very salty foods, and I started getting so depressed, this I also thought was normal.

Thin and exhausted, my relationship with my spouse strained. Weekends were a facade of energy, concealing the halted menstruation and pervasive exhaustion.

Gasping for breath during a short walk to the local market, a compassionate fishmonger came to my aid, driving me home. Neglecting my children, I found solace in a bed, drifting in and out of consciousness. A concerned friend intervened, arranging for an ambulance to take me to the town's infirmary.

Under the attentive care of a local doctor, I was diagnosed with a rare condition, secondary Addison disease. Monitored blood pressure and daily blood tests became routine. A relapse prompted screens around my bed, an additional saline drip, and the introduction of cortisone, marking a turning point in my recovery.

A month of recovery brought rest, walks, and adjustment to medication. Challenges with sodium digestion were eventually overcome, thanks to adjustments in dosage. Triumphantly, I emerged, my health seemingly under control. However, a minor setback occurred due to overwork, and years later, a recurrence traced back to the same disease required readmission to the local hospital. Treatment involving prednisone and Fludrocortisone, helped my low cortisol level and stabilized my sodium levels.

Through local care, understanding neighbors, and advancements in treatment, I triumphed over this disease, reclaiming my health and played many role as a loving mother and wife once again.

## Caregiver Perspectives in Addison's Disease

Caregiver perspectives in Addison's Disease offer a unique lens into the challenges and responsibilities accompanying the care of individuals with adrenal insufficiency.

## Key aspects of caregiver experiences include:

✓ **Vigilant Support:** Caregivers play a crucial role in providing vigilant support, particularly during adrenal crises or periods of illness. Their watchful presence ensures timely interventions and reinforces a safety net for those they care for.

✓ **Medication Management:** Caregivers are often actively involved in medication management, ensuring adherence to prescribed regimens. This involvement extends to understanding stress dosing principles and recognizing situations that may require adjustments in hormone replacement therapy.

✓ **Emotional Support:** Beyond the physical aspects, caregivers offer essential emotional support. Acknowledging the emotional impact of Addison's, they provide a listening ear, encouragement, and empathy, fostering a positive mental outlook for individuals with the condition.

✓ **Advocacy and Education:** Caregivers become advocates for individuals with Addison's, raising awareness within the broader community and healthcare settings. Their role includes educating others about the condition, reducing stigma, and facilitating understanding.

✓ **Emergency Preparedness:** Caregivers actively engage in emergency preparedness, understanding the importance of recognizing adrenal crises and implementing prompt interventions. Their proactive approach contributes to a sense of security for both the individual with Addison's and the caregiver themselves.

✓ **Balancing Care and Independence:** Striking a balance between providing necessary care and fostering independence is a delicate task for caregivers. Encouraging self-management while ensuring a safety net underscores the nuanced role they play.

✓ **Community Engagement:** Engaging with caregiver communities offers a valuable avenue for mutual support. Sharing experiences, tips, and strategies with other caregivers fosters a sense of solidarity and equips them with additional resources for optimal care.

Caregiver perspectives underscore the symbiotic relationship between caregivers and individuals with Addison's Disease. Their dedication, empathy, and advocacy significantly contribute to the well-being of those navigating the complexities of adrenal insufficiency, creating a supportive environment that enhances overall quality of life.

# Chapter eleven

# Appendix

## Glossary of Terms in Addison's Disease and Endocrinology

**Addison's Disease:** A chronic disorder characterized by the insufficient production of hormones, particularly cortisol and aldosterone, by the adrenal glands.

**Adrenal Crisis:** A life-threatening emergency caused by a severe deficiency of cortisol, often triggered by illness, trauma, or stress.

**Adrenal Glands:** Small glands located on top of each kidney responsible for producing essential hormones, including cortisol and aldosterone.

**Aldosterone:** A hormone produced by the adrenal glands that regulates salt and water balance in the body, crucial for maintaining blood pressure.

**Autoimmune Disease:** A condition where the immune system mistakenly attacks the body's own tissues; Addison's Disease is often caused by autoimmune destruction of the adrenal glands.

**Biomarkers:** Measurable substances in the body that indicate the presence of a disease or a specific physiological state. In Addison's, biomarkers may be explored for early detection.

**Corticosteroids:** Hormones, such as cortisol, produced by the adrenal glands that play a vital role in various physiological functions, including metabolism, immune response, and stress regulation.

**Electrolytes:** Essential minerals in the body, including sodium and potassium, which are regulated by aldosterone and impact various bodily functions, including nerve and muscle function.

**Endocrine System:** A complex network of glands and hormones that regulate numerous physiological processes, including metabolism, growth, and stress response.

**Genetic Predisposition:** An increased likelihood of developing a specific condition due to inherited genetic factors; certain genes are associated with an elevated risk of autoimmune disorders, including Addison's Disease.

**Hormone Replacement Therapy (HRT):** Treatment involving the administration of synthetic hormones, such as cortisol and aldosterone, to replace deficiencies in individuals with Addison's Disease.

**Hydrocortisone:** A synthetic form of cortisol commonly used in hormone replacement therapy for individuals with Addison's.

**Polyglandular Autoimmune Syndromes (APS):** A group of autoimmune disorders affecting multiple endocrine glands; Addison's Disease is often part of these syndromes.

**Precision Medicine:** An approach to medical treatment that considers individual differences in patients' genes, environments, and lifestyles, aiming for personalized and optimized care.

**Primary Addison's Disease:** Addison's resulting from a direct dysfunction or damage to the adrenal glands.

**Secondary Addison's Disease:** Addison's caused by a malfunction in the pituitary gland or hypothalamus, leading to insufficient stimulation of the adrenal glands.

**Stem Cell Therapy:** Investigational treatment involving the use of stem cells to regenerate damaged tissues, potentially offering new avenues for addressing adrenal tissue destruction in Addison's.

**Stress Dosing:** Adjusting hormone replacement therapy dosage during periods of stress, illness, or surgery to meet increased physiological demands and prevent adrenal crises.

**Telemedicine:** The use of telecommunications technology to provide medical care remotely, offering opportunities for regular check-ups and support for individuals with Addison's.

**Wearable Devices:** Technologies such as smartwatches or fitness trackers that can monitor and track various health parameters, potentially aiding in the continuous monitoring of cortisol levels in Addison's patients.

This glossary provides a foundation for understanding key terms related to Addison's Disease and endocrinology. As research and medical advancements progress, additional terms may emerge, further enriching our comprehension of this complex and dynamic field.

## Additional Resources for Addison's Disease Support and Information

Navigating life with Addison's Disease is aided by a wealth of resources offering support, education, and connection. Here are valuable sources for individuals, caregivers, and healthcare professionals:

**Patient Advocacy Organizations**
Organizations like the National Adrenal Diseases Foundation (NADF) and the Addison's Disease Self-Help Group (ADSHG) provide comprehensive information, support networks, and advocacy for individuals with Addison's.

## Medical Journals and Publications

Peer-reviewed journals such as the Journal of Clinical Endocrinology & Metabolism and Endocrine Practice publish research articles, clinical guidelines, and updates on Addison's Disease management.

## Online Forums and Communities

Platforms like Inspire or Reddit's Addison's Disease community offer spaces for individuals to share personal experiences, seek advice, and find a sense of community with others facing similar challenges.

## Telehealth Platforms

Telemedicine services, including platforms like Teladoc or Amwell, provide opportunities for virtual consultations, ensuring accessible and convenient healthcare, particularly for remote or homebound individuals.

## Educational Websites

Websites like the Mayo Clinic, WebMD, and MedlinePlus offer reliable information on Addison's Disease, its symptoms, diagnosis, and treatment options.

## Social Media Support Groups

Facebook groups and Twitter communities dedicated to Addison's Disease provide real-time interactions, facilitating global connections and immediate responses to queries.

**Books and Literature**
Written works such as "Living with Addison's Disease: A Guide for People with Addison's, Supporters, and Professionals" by Simon Pearce and "The Addisonian Crisis" by Charles S. Lieber offer in-depth insights into living with and managing Addison's.

**Counseling and Mental Health Resources**
Platforms like BetterHelp or psychology professionals with experience in chronic conditions can provide online counseling and support for addressing the mental health aspects of living with Addison's.

## Pharmacy Support Programs

Pharmacies and pharmaceutical companies often offer support programs providing information on medications, financial assistance, and access to educational materials for individuals on hormone replacement therapy.

**Endocrinology Clinics and Specialists**
Establishing a relationship with endocrinology clinics and specialists ensures access to up-to-date medical guidance and personalized care for Addison's Disease.
These additional resources create a robust network of support, information, and community for individuals and caregivers navigating the complexities of Addison's Disease. Regularly exploring and utilizing these avenues empowers individuals to stay informed, connected, and proactive in managing their health.

# Conclusion

Addison's Disease stands as a complex yet manageable challenge. As we conclude this exploration, it becomes evident that understanding, support, and resilience are pivotal components in the journey of those affected by this endocrine disorder.

Armed with a detailed comprehension of Addison's—from its nuanced symptoms to the intricacies of hormone replacement therapy—individuals, caregivers, and healthcare professionals are better equipped to navigate the complexities of this condition. The interplay between genetics, immunology, and hormonal balance becomes clearer, guiding the development of tailored treatment plans and paving the way for personalized care.

Personal stories, shared experiences, and caregiver perspectives add depth to our understanding. They illuminate the emotional impact, coping strategies, and triumphs in the face of adversity. The power of community, found in support groups and online forums, becomes a beacon of solidarity, offering comfort and encouragement.

Ongoing research endeavors and potential breakthroughs in immunomodulation, stem cell therapy, and precision medicine offer hope for more effective treatments and improved quality of life.

In the journey ahead, education remains a cornerstone. Empowering individuals with knowledge, advocating for increased awareness, and fostering a network of support create a foundation for resilience. From emergency preparedness to lifestyle adjustments, embracing a holistic approach to care ensures a well-rounded strategy for managing Addison's.